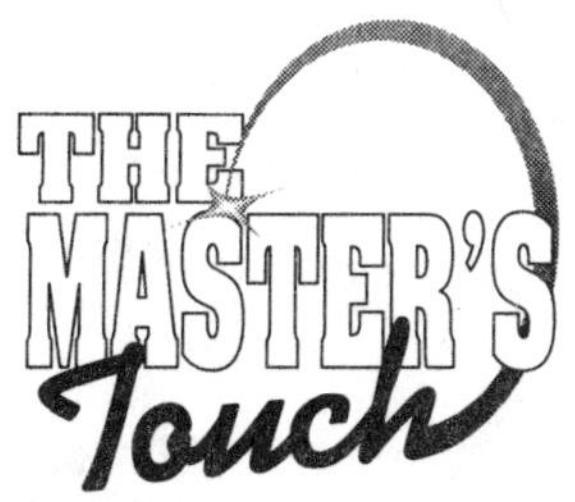

Living with Infertility

By Roger and Robin Sonnenberg

Edited by Thomas J. Doyle

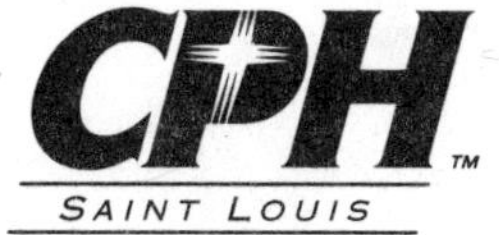

Editorial Assistant: Phoebe W. Wellman

3558 South Jefferson Avenue, St. Louis, MO 63118-3968
Manufactured in the United States of America

1 2 3 4 5 6 7 8 9 10 03 02 01 00 99 98 97 96 95 94

Contents

1 Stages

Focusing Our Sights

In this first session we will explore some of the common misconceptions about infertility as we discover the truth about infertility. We will then look at some biblical characters who struggled with infertility and discover truth from God's Word that confronts common misconceptions about infertility. Finally, we will search God's Word for comfort as we grieve over our struggle with infertility.

Focusing Our Attention

In my last year of college I fell in love with the most wonderful man in the world. We were both Christians. We both wanted the same things in life. We had everything planned out. After our education we would get married. We'd wait two to five years before we had children. By then we'd have a house and enough income. We were going to have two children—one boy and one girl—spaced two or three years apart. Everything else fell into place just as we wanted, except the children. . . . We were unable to have children as we had planned, not in the first five years or even in the next nine years. We discovered we were one of thousands of couples who would have to battle with the problem of infertility.

1. What plans do you remember making

with your spouse? Which dreams have been fulfilled? Which dreams are still unfulfilled?

2. Studies show infertility is on the rise. What might be the reason for this phenomenon?

Focusing on the Issue

Infertility? It's something very few people talk about, except if you are the one out of six couples who have a problem with infertility. Others may talk about it but with little understanding of the problem. They demonstrate their lack of knowledge about the subject in some of their comments:

- "Just get away for a week and you'll end up pregnant!"
- "If you need some instruction in the bedroom, I'll be happy to assist you."
- "Adopt a kid. Then you'll end up having a kid of your own."

In some respects, infertility might fall into the same category as the subject of sex. Though we live in an age of talk radio and tabloid television, where almost anything is discussed, people remain uninformed about infertility. Myths and misunderstandings of every nature surround the subjects of sex and infertility. Some of these myths about infertility only increase the struggle and hurts experienced by infertile couples. As you review the myths, check those you have dealt with personally.

___ **1. Infertility is a "female problem."** The causes for infertility can be in the woman, the man, a combination of both, or it can be of unknown etiology.

These are the primary causes of infertility in women:

- Infection leading to scarring and adhesions of the uterus, ovaries, or fallopian tubes
- Endometriosis, a sometimes painful condition in which cells from the uterine lining implant themselves outside the uterus, where they "bleed" at the time of menstruation, often causing ovarian cysts, scarring, and adhesions
- Irregular ovulation or anovulation (when ovulation fails to occur)
- Cervical infection, weakness, or blockage
- Uterine tumors, malformation, or extreme malpositioning of the uterus
- Hormonal deficiencies

The most frequent causes of infertility in men are azoospermia (the absence of sperm) or an inadequate number of sperm, motility (sperm swimming ability), or morphology (structure). Other causes of male infertility include the following:

- Sperm blockage, resulting from infection or a congenital defect
- Varicocele (varicose veins grouped in the scrotum)
- Undescended testicle
- Adult mumps
- Hormonal deficiencies
- Serious injury or accident affecting the reproductive organs
- Heat

___ **2. Infertility is something you simply have to accept because very little can be done about it.** Research over the last 10 years has made great strides in providing hope for many infertile couples.

___ **3. Infertility is a sexual problem.** The majority of infertile couples have the same normal sexual relations as fertile couples.

___ **4. Infertility is a psychological problem.** Up to 95 percent of infertile couples are unable to conceive because of physical problems. Needless to say, the very struggle over childlessness may produce psychological and emotional problems. Research has shown that couples who struggle with infertility go through stages of grief similar to those who experience the death of a loved one—stage 1: denial, stage 2: anger, stage 3: bargaining, stage 4: depression, stage 5: acceptance.

Focusing on the Word

Stories of infertility are sprinkled throughout Scripture—stories of couples agonizing over their childlessness. Sarah chose Hagar, her maidservant, as a surrogate to bear for her a child (Genesis 16:1–2). Hannah anguished over her childlessness and pleaded with God so fervently that she was accused of being drunk (1 Samuel 1:12–14).

1. Read about one couple's struggle with infertility as recorded in 1 Samuel 1:1–20. Identify some of the stages of grief experienced by Hannah and Elkanah.

❖❖❖❖❖❖❖❖❖❖❖❖❖❖❖❖❖❖❖❖❖❖❖❖❖❖❖❖❖❖❖❖

There was a certain man from Ramathaim, a Zuphite from the hill country of Ephraim, whose name was Elkanah son of Jeroham, the son of Elihu, the son of Tohu, the son of Zuph, an Ephraimite. He had two wives;

one was called Hannah and the other Peninnah. Peninnah had children, but Hannah had none.

Year after year this man went up from his town to worship and sacrifice to the LORD Almighty at Shiloh, where Hophni and Phinehas, the two sons of Eli, were priests of the Lord. Whenever the day came for Elkanah to sacrifice, he would give portions of the meat to his wife Peninnah and to all her sons and daughters. But to Hannah he gave a double portion because he loved her, and the LORD has closed her womb. And because the LORD had closed her womb, her rival kept provoking her in order to irritate her. This went on year after year. Whenever Hannah went up to the house of the LORD, her rival provoked her till she wept and would not eat. Elkanah her husband would say to her, "Hannah, why are you weeping? Why don't you eat? Why are you downhearted? Don't I mean more to you than ten sons?"

Once when they had finished eating and drinking in Shiloh, Hannah stood up. Now Eli the priest was sitting on a chair by the doorpost of the Lord's temple. In bitterness of soul Hannah wept much and prayed to the Lord. And she made a vow, saying, "O LORD Almighty, if You will only look upon Your servant's misery and remember me, and not forget Your servant but give her a son, then I will give him to the LORD for all the days of his life, and no razor will ever be used on his head."

As she kept on praying to the Lord, Eli observed her mouth. Hannah was praying in her heart, and her lips were moving but her voice was not heard. Eli thought she was drunk and said to her, "How long will you keep on getting drunk? Get rid of your wine."

"Not so, my lord," Hannah replied, "I am a woman who is deeply troubled. I have not been drinking wine or beer; I was pouring out my soul to the LORD. Do not take your servant for a wicked woman; I have been praying here out of my great anguish and grief."

Eli answered, "Go in peace, and may the God of Israel grant you what you have asked of Him."

She said, "May your servant find favor in your eyes." Then she went her way and ate something, and her face was no longer downcast.

Early the next morning they arose and worshiped before the LORD and then went back to their home at Ramah. Elkanah lay with Hannah his wife, and the Lord remembered her. So in the course of time Hannah conceived and gave birth to a son. She named him Samuel, saying, "Because I asked the LORD for him."

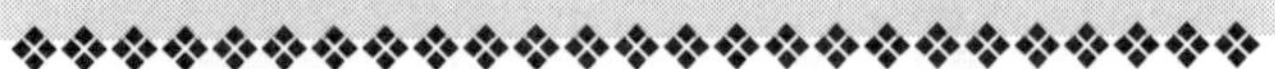

2. It is not unusual for childless couples to question God. In their questioning, they may blame God or even question whether or not they did something wrong, which brought God's disfavor upon them. This may lead them to bargain with the Lord, just as Hannah did (1 Samuel 1:10–11). What kinds of things might childless couples fear they are being punished for? How might infertile couples bargain with God?

3. Why is it easy for people to think they are being punished for some sin committed long ago?

"An eleven-year-old boy of my acquaintance was given a routine eye examination at school and found to be just nearsighted enough to require glasses. . . . The boy was deeply upset at the prospect, and would not tell anyone why. Finally one night as his mother was putting him to bed, the story came out. A week before the eye examination, the boy and two older friends were looking through a pile of trash that a neighbor had set out for collection, and found a copy *Playboy*. With a sense that they were doing something naughty, they spent several minutes looking at the pictures of unclothed women. When, a few days later, the boy failed the eye test at school and was found to need glasses, he jumped to the conclusion that God had begun the process of punishing him with blindness for looking at those pictures." (From When Bad Things Happen to Good People by Harold S. Kushner. Copyright 1981. Schocken Books, Inc.)

4. Quickly scan the Scriptures for a moment to see how childless couples may fear that barrenness is a punishment from God.

a. Who did Jacob blame for Rachel's barrenness (Genesis 30:1–3)?

b. What does Scripture give as the reason for Hannah's conception of Samuel (1 Samuel 1:19–20)?

c. The psalmist pictures children as "arrows" in Psalm 127:3–5. Why were children considered a blessing? (Note: the gate was the place where public business and litigation was done.)

Despite what it may seem like, barrenness is not a punishment for sin. As New Testament Christians we live under the banner of God's love and forgiveness because of the life, death, and resurrection of Jesus. Jesus died to forgive all of our sins. God does not use forgiven sins as an excuse to punish us.

5. Do you find any encouragement from Elkanah and Hannah to help you with your childlessness? Be specific.

Focusing on My Life

1. (Husbands) Have you ever felt like Elkanah, at times even getting angry because your wife seems to be obsessed with only one thing—to have a child (1 Samuel 1:8)? (Wives) Have you ever felt like your husband doesn't really understand how you feel about being childless?

2. In your struggle with infertility, have you found yourself questioning God with statements such as these?

❖❖❖❖❖❖❖❖❖❖❖❖❖❖❖❖❖❖❖❖❖❖❖❖❖❖❖❖❖❖❖❖

"Millie keeps having children, and she isn't even married. Why does God bless her with one child after another and us with none? She doesn't have adequate housing . . . can't provide them with even the basic needs . . . and yet she doesn't seem to have any trouble conceiving. Doesn't God care?"

"It's really disturbing to see many of the couples we've associated with for years divorcing. Most of them have children. Some day, God's going to have to answer to me why these divorced couples could have children and we, who have a solid and a good marriage, weren't able to have any children."

"Why does God allow a 16-year-old to become pregnant only to have her abort the baby?"

❖❖❖❖❖❖❖❖❖❖❖❖❖❖❖❖❖❖❖❖❖❖❖❖❖❖❖❖❖❖❖❖

3. How did God answer Job's questioning (Job 38:4–6, 22, 32)?

4. Circle the words(s) that best depict you at this time. **Denial,** *(The doctor doesn't know what he's talking about...)* **Anger,** *(You just don't understand what it's like!)* **Bargaining,** *(I'll be in church every Sunday if you'll only give me a child.)* **Depression,** *(It's no use...nothing will help!)* **Acceptance,** *(Okay, we've done everything we can. We've got to close this chapter in our lives.)*. During your struggle with infertility, what stages of grief have you experienced?

Jesus knows grief and struggle. He struggled before He made His final journey to the cross. He struggled because He took upon Himself the sins of the entire world—our sins of questioning and doubting, our sins of lovelessness and insensitivity toward one another. Jesus forgives these sins and offers help when we struggle—even when we struggle with infertility. No matter how much we grieve our situation, Jesus understands and promises to help.

> For we do not have a high priest who is unable to sympathize with our weakness, but we have One who has been tempted in every way, just as we are—yet was without sin. Let us then approach the throne of grace with confidence so that we may receive mercy and find grace to help us in our time of need. (Hebrews 4:15–16)

5. Knowing that God will give us "mercy and . . . grace to help us in our time of need" we can "approach the throne of grace with confidence." Choose a partner, preferably someone other than your spouse, and agree to be prayer partners. Share with this partner some of your grief and struggles. Ask your partner to pray that God would provide you with His comfort and strength. Remain prayer partners for the next five weeks, each week praying for different aspects of infertility, which we will discuss in the upcoming sessions.

Focusing on the Week Ahead

Write the words *Thy will be done* on an index card. Place the card somewhere in your home where you'll see it often. Talk to God about how you feel when you see the card, even if you're angry.

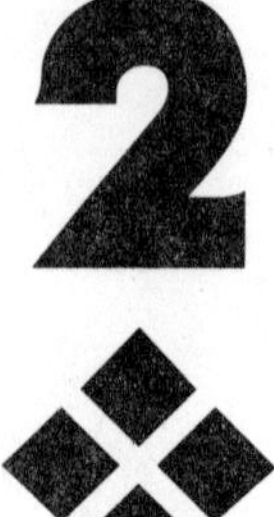

Coping

Focusing Our Sights

As we begin this session we will identify some of the questions and suggestions from well-meaning friends and relatives about our struggle with infertility. We will explore situations that challenge our ability to cope. Then we will identify that which enabled St. Paul to cope with struggles in his life. Finally, we will affirm the power of Jesus' love to strengthen and comfort us as we cope with the challenges infertility causes in our lives.

Focusing Our Attention

Every infertile couple has to deal with endless questions and suggestions from well-meaning friends and relatives. Read the following statements. How might you respond to these or similar statements?

1. "Isn't it about time you started having children?"

2. "Consider yourself fortunate you don't have any children. Ours have only brought us trouble!"

3. "Does your husband wear boxers or briefs? Guaranteed, if he wears briefs instead of boxers, you'll have a child in nine months."

4. "So you're one of those DINK (double income no kids) couples?"

Reread the statements. How might you lovingly, but honestly, respond to each?

Focusing on the Issue

Coping! It's one of the things infertile couples have to learn to do as they are bombarded with personal questions and examinations, requests and suggested solutions. Listen in on some of the comments shared by couples struggling with infertility:

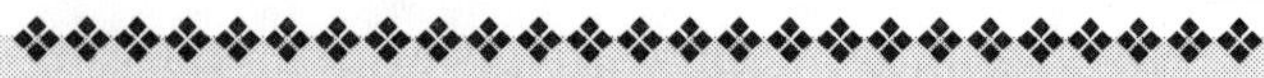

"I thought I was going to die when the nurse took the specimen bottle out of the bag and looked carefully at my sperm sample! I wanted to ask her what business it was of hers!"

"You think that's bad? You should be prodded and poked in the stirrups of the gynecologist's table. When I had my hysterosalpingogram, dye was injected into my uterus and the doctor, X-ray technician, and several other specialists watched on a closed-circuit television screen. Something so private seemed to be so public."

"I think the whole doctor's workup was invasive and embarrassing. 'How many times a week do you have sexual intercourse? What positions do you use when have sexual intercourse?' "

"I hate how our sex life has become programmed. It's lost spontaneity and intimacy. My wife has said to me more than a number of times, 'Honey, I'm sorry, I know you're tired, but we have to have sexual intercourse tonight. My temperature says so!' You try to explain that to someone and expect empathy? Forget it. My best friend said, 'Oh, boy, I wish I was that lucky!' "

"I hate it when people think our childlessness is a psychological or spiritual problem rather than a medical problem. My pastor says, 'Just pray about it.' He has no idea! He has six kids."

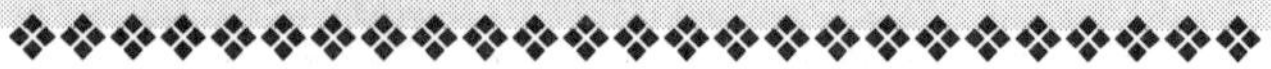

One survey shows that the following circumstances present some of the most challenging things infertile couples must cope with. Which of these have your experienced?

1. Surviving Mother's Day and Father's Day!

Special holidays and celebrations like Mother's Day and Father's Day can be extremely difficult. Without even thinking about hurting single people or infertile couples, churches often celebrate Mother's Day by giving each mother of the congregation corsages or some other special recognition. Even Christmas, a time when family celebrations are talked about and sung about, can be a time of emotional upheaval for a childless couple.

Have these special celebrations been difficult for you? If so, how have you handled these special days?

2. Surviving the reactions of insensitive, well-intentioned friends and relatives!

The reactions of people can vary. Your parents might constantly ask, "When are you going to give us a grandchild?" Others might say, "Just get away by yourselves for a while and everything will work out." Or, "Give up some of your work and you'll have children!" "Light some candles . . . take a bubble bath together . . . give each other a massage."

What kinds of things have people said to you that have been difficult for you to cope with?

3. Surviving the infertility workups!

Most infertile couples spend hours answering medical questions and meeting with fertility experts! What was once private becomes public. Everything is asked and nearly every part of the body is checked. All the while you're patiently waiting for the doctor in the waiting room, pregnant mothers march in and out of the office.

What has been the most difficult part of a doctor's workup for you and your spouse?

4. Surviving the feeling of isolation and low self-esteem.

It is not unusual for infertile couples to feel alone and out of the mainstream of the majority of couples their own age. The people you grew up with are having children, some even grandchildren, and you're still trying to have your first child. Often, a person's self-esteem can take a terrible hit when the doctor announces the reason for your infertility.

"I'll never forget when the doctor called both of us into his office. Both Darling and I had agreed that we wouldn't blame each other no matter what the doctor said. I delivered to the doctor's office several sperm specimens. My wife had all the basic workup. She always complained that men had it easy compared to women. I agreed with her until the doctor said, 'Tom, for whatever reason, it appears that you simply do not produce any sperm. We'll do further tests, but right now it doesn't look like you'll be able to father a child.' "

Later, in talking with some friends, the man explained that he and his wife were looking into adoption, because, as he said, "I shoot blanks." Though he said it in a joking manner, the man was hurting inside, feeling somewhat insecure in his masculinity.

Have you felt or do you feel isolated and out of the social mainstream because of your infertility? How has it affected your self-esteem?

5. Jot down some other special issues or difficult circumstances you've encountered in your struggle with infertility. Then compare your notes with the issues and circumstances of others in your group.

Focusing on God's Word

> To keep me from becoming conceited because of these surpassingly great revelations, there was given me a thorn in my flesh, a messenger of Satan, to torment me. Three times I pleaded with the Lord to take it away from me. But He said to me, "My grace is sufficient for you, for My power is made perfect in weakness." (2 Corinthians 12:7–9)

Almost every Christian can point to some "thorn in the flesh," physical or psychological, from which he has prayed to be released, but hasn't found the release he's prayed for.

1. How did St. Paul's thorn affect his life

2. In his human weakness, what did Paul discover?

3. Does your infertility often feel like a "thorn" that torments you? Explain.

4. How do you respond to the Lord's words to Paul?

What, then, shall we say in response to this? If God is for us, who can be against us? He who did not spare His own Son, but gave Him up for us all—how will He not also, along with Him, graciously give us all things? (Romans 8:31–32)

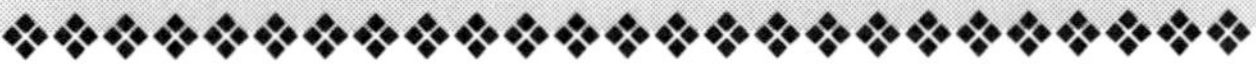

5. According to Romans 8:32, what did God do to care for our greatest weakness—sin?

6. If He "did not spare His own Son, but gave Him up for us all" what else can we be assured He will do for us, including help in coping with the anguish of infertility?

Focusing on My Life

Of the challenges of infertility discussed earlier, which do you have most difficulty dealing with (rank the most difficult with a 1 and the least difficult with a 5)?

_____1. Surviving Mother's Day and Father's Day!

_____2. Surviving the reactions of insensitive, well-intentioned friends and relatives!

_____3. Surviving the infertility workups!

_____4. Surviving the feeling of isolation and low self-esteem.

_____5. Other

Write Romans 8:32 and the following on an index card: *"He who did not spare His own Son, but gave Him up for us all—how will He not also, along with Him, graciously give us all things," including my surviving.*

____

Post it in a place where you will see it often.

Focusing on the Week Ahead

Satan wants us to believe that we're alone in coping with our problems, including the problem of infertility. However, God is not dead! Jesus lives, and we are not left alone to cope with the problems of life! This week, when you get discouraged and are tempted to believe that you're alone, examine the following Scripture passages: **Romans 8:37; Philippians 4:13; Ephesians 3:14–16; 2 Peter 1:4;** and **1 Corinthians 10:13.**

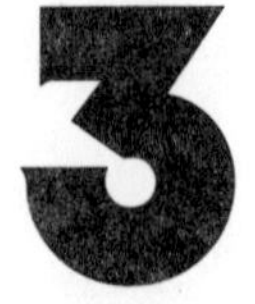

Hoping

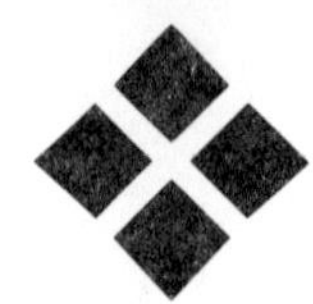

Focusing Our Sights

In this session we will define hope as it relates to the lives of Christians. We will then explore the story of Abraham and Sarah, who remained hopeful in spite of a situation most would consider hopeless. Finally, we will examine God's promises. His promises give us hope in the midst of hopelessness, they affirm the power of His love for us in Christ.

Focusing Our Attention

A woman with very little income other than her social security check religiously bought a lottery ticket every week.

One of her neighbors criticized her saying, "With as little money as you have, why would you waste a dollar each week on a lottery ticket?"

The woman replied, "I think it's worth it. That $1 lottery ticket gives me a whole week's hope!"

1. What kind of hope did the lottery ticket give the woman each week?

In a survey, couples shared that they tried some of the following remedies—lost weight; stopped drinking alcohol; took warm, even cold showers instead of hot showers; tried different positions when making love; crawled down the hallway on all fours after making love pushing a peanut with one's nose; laid with pillows under the wife's knees after making love—hoping the remedies would help them have a child.

2. List some suggestions you have received in order to help you conceive? Did you take any of the suggestions seriously? If so, why did you? If not, why not?

3. Someone said, "You can live for several weeks without food, a few days without water, about eight minutes without air, but not a minute without hope." How does hope play an important part in your struggle with infertility?

Focusing on the Issue

The true stories of three couples reflect the emotional roller coaster many infertile couples ride as they hope for a child.

For seven years Larry and Meagan tried to have a child. Finally, they went to an infertility specialist. The medical workups proved to be much more expensive than either had expected. Larry's sperm sample showed a high sperm count and normal sperm activity. Meagan's physical and laboratory workups included a hysterosalpingogram (X-rays are taken as a dye is injected into the uterus and the Fallopian tubes to see if there are any blockages), an endometrial biopsy (uterine lining is taken from the uterus to see if implantation of the embryo can take place), and a test for endometriosis (uterine tissue found growing outside the uterus and blocking the reproductive tract). Meagan's tests indicated that there were no apparent biological reasons why she should not be able to conceive.

The doctor put Meagan on Clomid, a mild fertility drug, for a period of six months. At the end of six months, Meagan was still not pregnant. The doctor then suggested in vitro fertilization (IVG) or the Gamete intrafallopian transfer (GIFT) program.

In in vitro fertilization the eggs of the woman and the sperm of the man are mixed outside the body in a petri dish and then placed back into the uterus, where, hopefully, implantation will take place. In the GIFT program, sperm and eggs are mixed outside the body and are placed back into the natural environment, the Fallopian tube, in order to fertilize.

The cost for either of the two procedures is approximately $3,000–$7,000. Larry and Meagan had exhausted all their savings. Neither of their parents were willing to loan them the money. Meagan's parents stated, "Just trust God. Remember, when you're at the end of your rope, He is just at the beginning of His."

1. What do you think Larry and Meagan should do?

a. Get the money they need so that they can know in their hearts that they have done everything possible to have a child.

b. Tell their parents, "You're right. We do need to trust God more!"

c. Give up trying to have a child of their own and turn their attention to other worthwhile causes such as feeding the hungry or becoming foster parents.

d. Confront Meagan's parents.

e. Other ______________________________

____

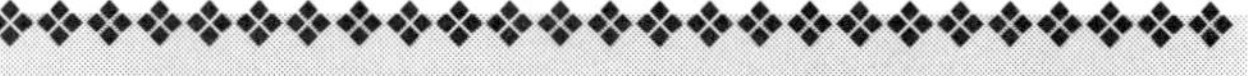

Don and Sandy were childless the first years of their marriage. After consulting infertility specialists, the only thing that could be determined was that Sandy had a mild case of endrometriosis. She underwent surgery to correct the endrometriosis and shortly afterward became pregnant. Kevin was born.

For the next three years they tried to have a second child, but to no avail. They returned to the same infertility specialist, and Sandy once again underwent surgery to get rid of the endometriosis, which had returned. This time, unlike the first time, Sandy did not get pregnant immediately afterward. She and her husband joined the ranks of many couples who suffer from wanting a second child but are unable to conceive. This phenomenon is called "secondary infertility."

Don and Sandy sought support by joining a special support group for infertile couples, but they often got the impression from others in the group that they really shouldn't be complaining. After all, they did have one child, and many of the couples didn't have any. Even when they went to their pastor, he denied them the opportunity to talk about what they were feeling by asking them to count their blessings and talk about the child they did have. They felt isolated, and they buried their feelings.

2. What do you think Don and Sandy should do?

a. "Count their blessings" just like the pastor said, and stop complaining.

b. Go to another infertility specialist and go through the medical workups once again.

c. Look into adoption.

d. Find couples who are also going through "secondary infertility" and form their own support group.

e. Other ______________________________

____

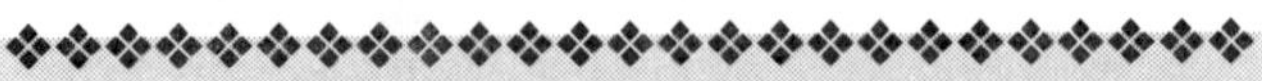

It was determined immediately in Jose and Cindy's case that Jose's sperm count was low. He was put on medication in hopes that the count would rise, but to no avail. He gave up drinking alcohol, started wearing shorts rather than briefs, took warm rather than hot showers, but nothing seemed to help. The doctor told them that if they hoped to have a child, a donor's sperm would need to be injected into Cindy during ovulation. Jose's friends thought Jose and Cindy were crazy for even contemplating such a program. Though Jose and Cindy wanted a child, they feared that using this method may not be God-pleasing.

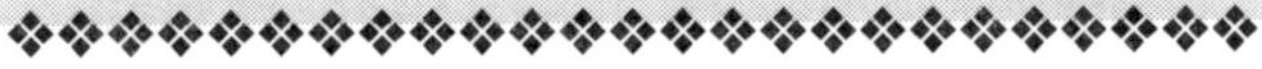

3. What do you think Jose and Cindy should do?

a. Listen to their friends and not even contemplate such a program.

b. Seek counsel from their pastor or other trusted Christian friends regarding the ethical ramifications of this procedure.

c. Seek to adopt a child.

d. Go for the artificial insemination, choosing a donor who is most like Jose.

e. Other ______________________________

____

The descriptions of these three couples give only a micropicture of the ups and downs of couples who struggle with infertility. The reason each of the couples spent endless hours in a doctor's office or thousands of dollars is simple—each couple wanted a child. Only those who have experienced the pain of infertility can understand it fully. They hoped each procedure and each new specialist would enable them to have their own child.

Focusing on God's Word

One of the ways many infertile couples find help is by meeting with other infertile couples. Suppose you met a couple by the name of Abraham and Sarah who struggled with infertility. Review their story from the selected verses of Genesis 15–21. Then answer the questions.

The word of the LORD came to Abram in a vision: "Do not be afraid, Abram. I am your shield, your very great reward."

But Abram said, "O Sovereign LORD:, what can You give me since I remain childless and the one who will inherit my estate is Eliezer of Damascus?" And Abram said, "You have given me no children; so a servant in my household will be my heir."

Then the word of the LORD came to him, "This man will not be your heir, but a son coming from your own body will be your heir." He took him outside and said, "Look up at the heavens and count the stars—if indeed you can count them." Then He said to him, "So shall your offspring be."

Abram believed the LORD, and He credited it to him as righteousness. . . .

Now Sarai, Abram's wife, had borne him no children. But she had an Egyptian maidservant named Hagar; so she said to Abram, "The LORD has kept me from having children. Go, sleep with my maidservant; perhaps I can build a family through her."

Abram agreed to what Sarai said. So after Abram had been living in Canaan ten years, Sarai his wife took her Egyptian maidservant Hagar and gave her to her husband to be his wife. He slept with Hagar, and she conceived. . . .

When Abram was ninety-nine years old, the LORD appeared to him and said, "I am God Almighty; walk before Me and be blameless. I will confirm My covenant between Me and you and will greatly increase your numbers." . . .

God also said to Abraham, "As for Sarai your wife, you are no longer to call her Sarai; her name will be Sarah. I will bless her and will surely give you a son by her. I will bless her so that she will be the mother of nations; kings of peoples will come from her."

Abraham fell facedown; he laughed and said to himself, "Will a son be born to a man a hundred years old? Will Sarah bear a child at the age of ninety?" And Abraham said to God, "If only Ishmael might live under your blessing!" . . .

Then the LORD said, "I will surely return to you about this time next year, and Sarah your wife will have a son."

Now Sarah was listening at the entrance to the tent, which was behind him. Abraham and Sarah were already old and well advanced in years, and Sarah was past the age of childbearing. So Sarah laughed to herself as she thought, "After I am worn out and my master is old, will I now have this pleasure?"

Then the LORD said to Abraham, "Why did Sarah laugh and say, 'Will I really have a child, now that I am old?' Is anything too hard for the LORD? I will return to you at the appointed time next year and Sarah will have a son."

Sarah was afraid, so she lied and said, "I did not laugh."

But He said, "Yes, you did laugh." . . .

Now the LORD was gracious to Sarah as He had said, and the LORD did for Sarah what He had promised. Sarah became pregnant and bore a son to Abraham in his old age, at the very time God had promised him. Abraham gave the name Isaac to the son Sarah bore him. When his son Isaac was eight days old, Abraham circumcised him, as God commanded him. Abraham was a hundred years old when his son Isaac was born to him.

Sarah said, "God has brought me laughter, and everyone who hears about this will laugh with me." And she added, "Who would have said to Abraham that Sarah would nurse children? Yet I have borne him a son in his old age."

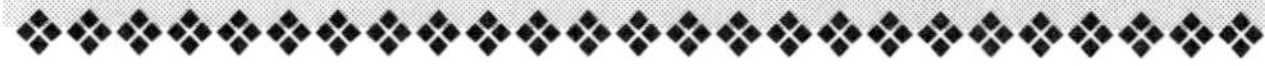

1. Why would Abraham and Sarah make a great couple with whom to discuss infertility (Genesis 15:2–3)?

2. A concern voiced by many older couples seeking to have children is that they're getting older every day and that their biological clocks are running out. Yet how old were Abraham and Sarah when they finally had a child (Genesis 17:17–19)?

3. In what ways do Abraham and Sarah mirror some of the frustrations and desperate means infertile couples will go through in order to have children (Genesis 16:1–4)?

4. Review Genesis 17:15–18 and 18:10–15. Do you think Abraham and Sarah's laughter was excusable? Why?

5. In Hebrews 11 Abraham is described as one who was "sure of what [he] hope[d] for and certain of what [he could] not see" (Hebrews 11:1). In whom did Abraham trust?

Focusing on My Life

1. On the following continuum, rank your hope of having a child. Explain your answer to the person next to you.

1 ______________________________ 10

(No longer hopeful) (Very hopeful)

2. What one thing do you fear more than anything?

___ a. My biological time clock is running out!

___ b. We have become so focused on having children that our marriage is hurting.

___ c. If something doesn't happen soon, I'm afraid I'm going to have a nervous breakdown.

___ d. We will never have a child.

___ e. Other ______________________________

____

3. What kind of circumstances have made you laugh as you have struggled with infertility? How has laughter helped you deal with the problem of infertility over the years?

4. Read slowly Isaiah 40:31–32.

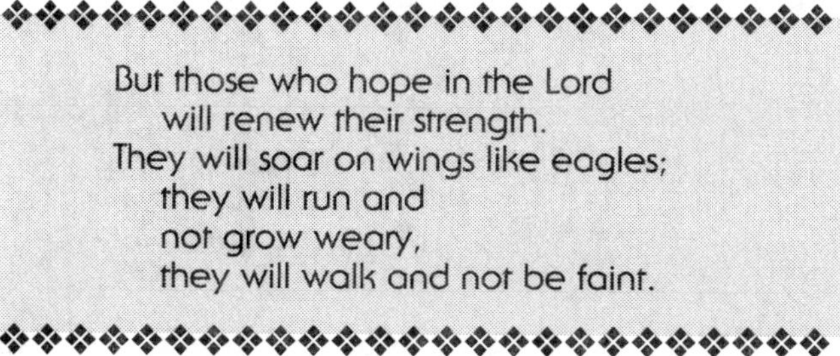

But those who hope in the Lord
  will renew their strength.
They will soar on wings like eagles;
  they will run and
  not grow weary,
  they will walk and not be faint.

Isaiah reminds us to "hope in the LORD" (40:31). This is not "wishful anticipating." It is trusting in God, who never disappoints. To "renew" means literally to "exchange strength." We hope in the Lord as we study and meditate on His Holy Word. In doing so, we exchange our weakness for God's great strength. As Christians, Jesus clothes us with His righteousness; He exchanges His holiness for our sinfulness. He clothes us with new hope! New tomorrows.

Pray together:

Lord God, the promise is ours: "But those who hope in the LORD will renew their strength" (Isaiah 40:31).

So come, take our despair and turn it into hope; Take our weakness and give us Your strength, knowing that whatever tomorrow may bring us, we are Yours through the blood of Jesus and the promise is ours:

"[*We*] *will soar on wings like eagles;*
[*we*] *will run and not grow weary,*
[*we*] *will walk and not be faint"* (Isaiah 40:31).

In the Name of Jesus. Amen.

Focusing on the Week Ahead

Copy **Isaiah 40:30–31** on an index card and post it where you and your spouse will see it often, such as, on your bathroom mirror! You might even want to commit these verses to memory for those times when you need to be reminded of God's promise of hope.

4 Seeking

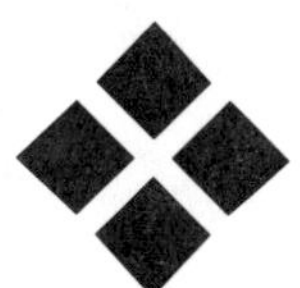

Focusing Our Sights

In this session we will examine current ways in which couples seek help for their infertility. We will then use God's Word as the guide by which we determine whether or not a method for dealing with infertility is God pleasing. We will explore how Jesus can help a couple struggling with infertility. Finally, we will affirm the power of Jesus' love to give hope and comfort to lives troubled by infertility.

Focusing Our Attention

In 1993 the story about a little girl named Jessica touched the world. Given up by her biological mother at the time of birth, Jessica lived for two years with Jan and Roberta DeBoer, a printer and a homemaker, who for two years tried to adopt her. They gave her everything a little girl would want. Then one day the unspeakable seemed to happen: the Michigan Supreme Court ruled that Jan and Roberta DeBoer had to give Jessica back to Dan and Cara Schmidt, the biological parents.

The story affected more than the two sets of parents, involved directly. It affected thousands of adoptive parents in the U.S., too. They wondered whether their adopted children might be taken from their homes by a seemingly insensitive legal social services system. For the thousands considering adoption, fear made them step back and ask whether they wanted to risk such terrible grief.

The case of baby Jessica—and similar cases in recent years—raises many legal and ethical questions about adoption, including the following:

1. Agree or disagree. Due process and the rights of biological parents are just as important as the well-being of a child, the rights of the adopting parents, or the relationship the adopting parents have developed with a child (and/or vice versa).

2. Agree or disagree. It is more important for a child to grow up in its biological family—even if the family situation is troubled or unstable—than it is for a child to be raised by an adopting family, even if that family can offer the child a more stable and less-troubled environment.

3. Agree or disagree. Adoption should benefit the child; adoption should not be viewed as a convenience for infertile couples.

4. Agree or disagree. Adopted children have a right to know who their biological parents are, and to reject their adopting family.

Focusing on the Issue

Adoption is one of many solutions for infertile couples. For others, adoption is not a viable option. The methods of resolution for infertility vary from individual to individual, from couple to couple. Listed are some of the most common ways childless couples seek help for their infertility.

Treating Male Infertility

Though medical research is rapidly advancing in this area, there is still much to be

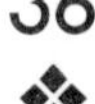

discovered in treating male infertility, especially when a male has a low or no sperm count.

Treating Female Infertility

Depending on the nature of the problem, great advances have been made in the area of treating female infertility. Through either surgery or medical treatment, many childless couples have been helped.

Artificial Insemination

In Vitro Fertilization (IVF), Gamete Intrafallopian Transfer (GIFT), and Tubal Ovum Transfer

In vitro fertilization has also been termed the "test-tube baby" solution, since eggs and sperm are placed in a petri dish and allowed to fertilize before placing the fertilized ovum back in the woman's uterus. The gamete intrafallopian transfer (GIFT) is a procedure in which the sperm and eggs are mixed outside the body but are placed in the fallopian tube to fertilize rather than in a sterile dish.

In a tubal ovum transfer, an egg is retrieved and transferred past the damaged parts of the fallopian tubes, where it is fertilized either by regular intercourse or artificial insemination.

Adoption

To adopt is often one solution considered by infertile couples at one time or another. Well-meaning friends will even suggest that adoption is a means of curing infertility; "Just adopt and then you'll have a biological child of your own." Statistics, however, do not substantiate this premise.

Surrogate Motherhood

There are advertisements in many major newspapers that identify women who for a fee will agree to bear a child for an infertile couple. Throughout its history, the program has raised its share of complications and ethical questions. For example, some surrogate mothers have refused to relinquish their children once they've been born. Some see this practice as nothing more than a means of selling and buying babies.

As you review the list, categorize which procedures you think are acceptable for a couple to use? Which procedures do you feel are questionable practices for a Christian? Which are not acceptable for a Christian? Explain the reason for your answers.

Acceptable Procedures	Questionable Procedures	Unacceptable Procedures

Focusing on God's Word

Read each of the following Scripture passages. Underline words and/or phrases that speak to the ways childless couples can get help for their infertility (review "Focusing on the Issue"). Based on these passages, we can determine a number of things concerning God's will for childless couples seeking to have a child.

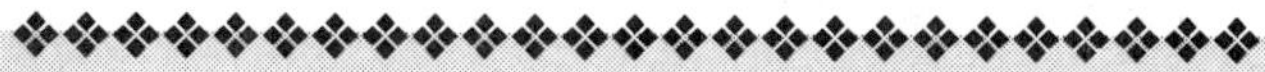

God blessed them [the newly created man and woman] and said to them, "Be fruitful and increase in number; fill the earth and subdue it. Rule over the fish of the sea and the birds of the air and over every living creature that moves on the ground." (Genesis 1:28)

So the LORD God caused the man to fall into a deep sleep; and while he was sleeping, He took one of the man's ribs and closed up the place with flesh. Then the LORD God made a woman from the rib He had taken out of the man, and He brought her to the man.

The man said, "This is now bone of my bones and flesh of my flesh; she shall be called 'woman,' for she was taken out of man."

For this reason a man will leave his father and mother and be united to his wife, and they will become one flesh.

The man and his wife were both naked, and they felt no shame. (Genesis 2:21–25)

Remember that You molded me like clay. Will You now turn me to dust again? Did You not pour me out like milk and curdle me like cheese, clothe me with skin and flesh and knit me together with bones and sinews? You gave me life and showed me kindness, and in Your providence watched over my spirit. (Job 10:9–12)

For You created my inmost being; You knit me together in my mother's womb. I praise You because I am fearfully and wonderfully made; Your works are wonderful, I know that full well. My frame was not hidden from You when I was made in the secret place. When I was woven together in the depths of the earth, Your eyes saw my unformed body. All the days ordained for me were written in Your book before one of them came to be. (Psalm 139:13–17)

1. Based on these passages write as many statements as possible about life and its beginnings.

2. How might these passages assist you as you consider

- in vitro fertilization using the husband's sperm

- in vitro fertilization using a donor's sperm

- gamete intrafallopian transfer using the husband's sperm

• gamete intrafallopian transfer using a donor's sperm

• adoption

• surrogate motherhood

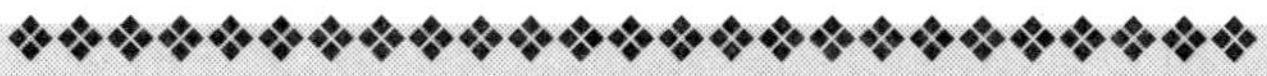

In the 1980s a standing committee of the Division of Theological Studies of the Lutheran Council in the U.S.A., after a two-year discussion, published its findings. . . . While The Lutheran Church—Missouri Synod has not established an official position on IVF [In Vitro Fertilization], the participants from the LCMS concurred: "IVF does not *in and of itself* violate the will of God as reflected in the Bible, when the wife's egg and the husband's sperm are used." The LCMS participants concluded that IVF is unobjectionable however, only when it is carried out subject to two limitations:

a. Because the Biblical injunction to be fruitful and multiply was given by God to a man and a woman united in the one-flesh union of marriage . . . , only the sperm and the eggs of a man and woman united in marriage may be employed. Any use of donor sperm or eggs involves the intrusion of a third party into the one-flesh union and is contrary to the will of God. For the same reason surrogate wombs may not be used.

b. Because the unborn are persons in God's sight from the time of conception . . . , *all* fertilized eggs must be returned to the womb of the woman. Any experimentation with, destruction of, or storage of unneeded or defective fertilized eggs fails to accord respect and reverence for new life brought into being by God at the moment of conception and is, therefore, contrary to His will. The same considerations preclude any required agreement of the woman to permit the interruption of an IVF pregnancy for any reason other than to prevent her death. (From *Life Choices: Who Decides? Following God's Word in Life and Death Decisions* by John Klotz. Copyright 1991 by Concordia Publishing House. All rights reserved.)

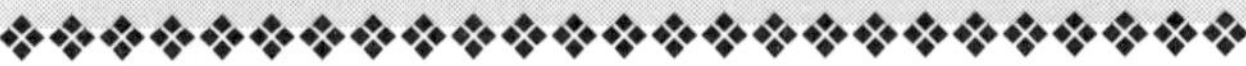

3. React to the quote from *Life Choices: Who Decides?*

Focusing on My Life

1. Couples contemplating treatments for infertility must consider a number of important factors. Which of the following factors are most pressing for you now?

__ a. The cost of a treatment

__ b. The Word of God concerning the possible treatments

__ c. The success rate of a treatment

__ d. The emotional roller-coaster ride of each new treatment

__ e. The danger of the procedure (e.g., the biological parents changing their minds in an adoption)

__ f. All of the above

__ g. Other______________________________

2. How are you allowing God to help you with your fears? Have you allowed the Holy Spirit, working through God's Word, to help you make the right decision about which program or treatment might be best for you and your spouse? Have you prayed about it together? Has today's study caused you to have any second thoughts about methods used to overcome infertility?

At this time you might feel guilt—guilt over past choices and decisions or about decisions and choices you have considered. Remember Jesus' death on the cross was the once-for-all sacrifice for *all* sins. He eagerly forgives repentant sinners for all of the times they have failed to consult His Word or ignored His Word when making difficult decisions.

If we claim to be without sin, we deceive ourselves and the truth is not in us. If we confess our sins, He is faithful and just and will forgive us our sins and purify us from all unrighteousness. If we claim we have not sinned, we make Him out to be a liar and His Word has no place in our lives.

My dear children, I write this to you so that you will not sin. But if anybody does sin, we have one who speaks to the Father in our defense—Jesus Christ, the Righteous One. He is the atoning sacrifice for our sins, and not only for ours but also for the sins of the whole world. (1 John 1:8–2:2)

Pray together:

Father, how great a love You have "lavished on us, that we should be called children of God" (1 John 3:1). Our thanks.

Father, "when the time had fully come, [You] sent [Your] Son, born of a woman, born under law, to redeem those [of us] under law, that we might receive the full rights of sons" (Galatians 4:4–5). Our thanks.

Father, You have made us "heir[s]" of all You possess (Galatians 4:7). Our thanks.

Important! Special! That's who we are! Your sons and daughters. As we struggle over our infertility, no one else may fully understand, but we know You do. Our thanks.

And yes, You not only understand, but You continue to help and guide us as we seek to have a child. Our thanks.

Amen.

Focusing on the Week Ahead

Go to your local library and research some of the newest techniques and procedures that are used to help infertile couples. Plan to share interesting information at the beginning of the next session.

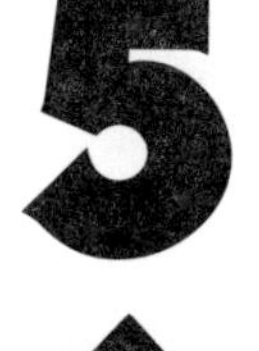

Moving On

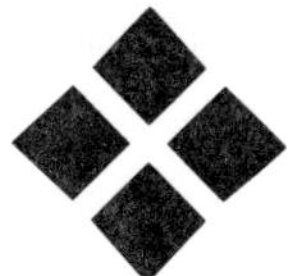

Focusing Our Sights

In this session we will examine the importance of closing the infertility chapter in our life so we can move ahead with the next chapter of our lives. Then we will search God's Word for advice and assistance as we prepare to move on. Finally we will develop a plan to continue to serve God as we move ahead with our lives.

Focusing Our Attention

Surveys have shown that infertility can place a tremendous strain on a marriage. The infertility issue can often uncover or magnify other problems in a marriage.

"This baby business has taken over our lives. All she ever talks about is having babies."

"Sex isn't spontaneous and fun anymore. It's something we do according to the chart whether we want to or not."

"As hard as I try to understand, she says I'm insensitive to how she feels."

1. How can infertility strain a marriage?

2. For what other reasons, other than for the sake of their marriage, is it important for couples to close the chapter on infertility?

Focusing on the Issue

Each couple must decide when to write the final pages to their chapter on infertility and to move on with the rest of life. There is a time when a couple can no longer think about temperature charts, the timing of sexual intercourse, or take one more emotional roller coaster ride with another procedure, only to discover pregnancy did not occur. For one couple, it might be when the third infertility specialist has just told them, "Your infertility tests show clearly that you will not be able to conceive a child. Even if you do, you will not be able to carry the baby to full term." For another couple, it might be after trying in vitro fertilization several times and after depleting their savings account. Whenever that time comes, it is important to close the chapter *together* and move on *together*. It means making a decision to change one's focus and to make plans for the future that may look somewhat different than the original plan. It will be a time when you stop dwelling on the whys! As a couple closes the chapter, it is important they consider the following things:

1. What has infertility done to your marriage over the years? Has it brought you closer together? Has it pushed you apart? Do you need to regroup as a husband and wife in order to move forward? Would it be helpful to seek some professional Christian counseling?

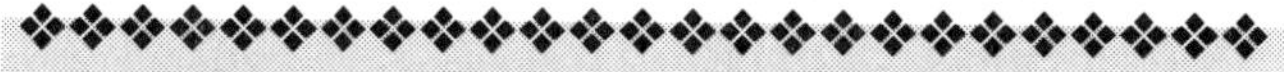

In words that many infertile couples will find affirming, the late Christian counselor Walter Trobisch addressed childless marriages. Speaking to an African audience, he quoted Genesis 2:24, "Therefore, a man leaves his father and his mother and cleaves to his wife and they become one flesh." Trobisch then asked how this verse ends, and a man replied, "With a full stop," or period. Trobisch emphasized this "full stop," noting that in that key verse about marriage, a verse quoted four times in the Bible, there is not a word about children. "The effect of these words on my audience was tremendous," he recalled. It was as if I had thrown a bomb into the church." For in the culture of those to whom he was speaking barrenness is sufficient grounds for divorce. "Don't misunderstand me," he continued. "Children are a blessing of God. The Bible emphasizes this over and over again . . . Children are a blessing to marriage, but they are an additional blessing to marriage. When God created Adam and Eve, he blessed them and then he said to them: 'Be fruitful and multiply.' From the Hebrew text it is clear that this commandment was an additional action to the action of blessing. Therefore, when the Bible describes the indispensable elements of marriage, it is significant that children are not expressly mentioned. Leaving, cleaving, and becoming one flesh are sufficient. Full stop . . . The full stop means that the child does not make marriage a marriage. A childless marriage is also a marriage in the full sense of the word."

(Excerpts taken from *Without Child: A Compassionate Look at Infertility*, © 1990 by Martha G. Stout. Used by permission of Harold Shaw Publishers, Wheaton, IL. [Primary source: Walter Trobisch, *I Married You* (San Francisco: Harper & Row, 1971), 20–21.])

2. Remember, a family can be two people! We're not less because we're only two. As Christians we are members of a large family—God's family.

The next time someone asks if you have a family, what will you say?

3. Being childless is not the end of the world. There is a loss without children but never a loss that doesn't open up new opportunities. God has many unique ministries for people other than parenting. Every person has been given something by God to benefit others and glorify Him.

Someone said, "He who fails to plan, plans to fail." How about making some plans to provide some surrogate mothering or fathering? Think of ways you can touch the lives of others in the things you say and do. Think of people in your life who were single, or married, and never had any children. How have they played a profound role in your life? Could it be that God has called you to be such a person for some child or children? Your godchildren? Your nieces or nephews? Sunday school students? (Continue to stretch your imagination . . . providing a home for an unwed mother . . . foster parenting.)

Warning: Coping with infertility can bring about strange over-compensation at times. For example, one childless woman became the great animal savior of her community. Every stray dog and cat became a welcome guest at her home. She spent excessive time caring for these stray animals, often ignoring her own husband.

List some other things couples will need to do in order to close the chapter of life entitled "Infertility":

Focusing on God's Word

> One thing I do: Forgetting what is behind and straining toward what is ahead, I press on toward the goal to win the prize for which God has called me heavenward in Christ Jesus. (Philippians 3:13–14)

1. What good advice does St. Paul give us in these verses?

2. We are called to forget! Before we can forget, however, we need to know we are forgiven! Do we need forgiveness for being insensitive at times to our spouse's needs and cries? To whom must we go first for this forgiveness (John 1:29; 1 Peter 2:24)?

3. Underline the word(s) from Philippians 3:13–14 that indicates that life ahead may not be easy.

4. What is the ultimate prize for the Christian?

5. How does the "prize" enable you to strain toward what is ahead?

6. Although the future is uncertain, what promise of God is certain?

Focusing on My Life

1. Is it time for you to close the chapter on infertility in your life, or if not now, when?

2. As difficult as moving forward may be, what promise does the psalmist give you?

God is our refuge and strength,
an ever-present help in trouble.
Therefore we will not fear, though the earth give way
and the mountains fall into the heart of the sea,
though its waters roar and foam
and the mountains quake with their surging.

(Psalm 46:1–3)

3. What can I do to help my spouse move forward?

____ a. Listen more

____ b. Never talk about babies again

____ c. Do some dreaming and future planning together

____ d. Seek counseling together

____ e. Other______________________________

____

____

4. The Scriptures remind us that we should "encourage one another and build each other up" (1 Thessalonians 5:11). How can we as a church help childless couples?

____ a. Provide support groups for them

____ b. Ask them to help staff the nursery

____ c. Never say a word to them about babies

____ d. Set up surrogate parenting and grandparenting programs in the church

____ e. Other______________________________

____

____

5. David gives us a positive action in the face of childlessness. When he heard his child had died, Scripture tells us:

Then David got up from the ground. After he had washed, put on lotions and changed his clothes, he went into the house of the LORD and worshiped. Then he went to his own house, and at his request they served him food, and he ate. (2 Samuel 12:20)

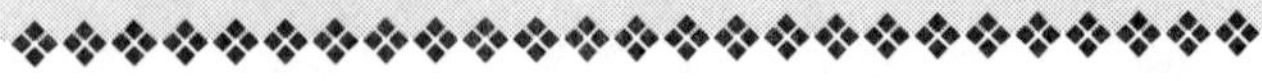

When and if the time comes for you to close the chapter on infertility, it will not be easy. But the God who created you, redeemed you with the precious blood of His Son, Jesus Christ, and brought you to faith through the power of the Holy Spirit will also sustain you and make it possible for you to move forward.

Focusing on the Week Ahead

Spend some time this week thanking God for each member of the group who participated with you in this special Bible study. Remember to continue to pray for the special concerns of these couples with whom you have so intimately shared over the last few weeks. Try to stay in touch with each other. Jot a note to each other periodically. Telephone one another. Remember each other during especially difficult times—Mother's Day or after hearing someone's $7,000 in vitro fertilization didn't work.

Notes for the Leader

1—Stages

❖ Focusing Our Sights

(About 2 minutes.) Read aloud the opening paragraph.

❖ Focusing Our Attention

(About 5 minutes.) Ask a volunteer to read aloud the opening quote. Discuss the questions.

1. Answers will vary.

2. Infertility is on the rise for a number of reasons. Couples are waiting longer before they get married. As they get older they become less fertile. Use of drugs and alcohol can also alter the sperm count or the eggs. The rise of diseases such as gonorrhea, chlamydia, and syphilis have also brought about a rise in infertility.

❖ Focusing on the Issue

(About 20 minutes.) Ask for volunteers to read aloud the opening paragraphs. Then review the myths listed, asking the participants to check those they personally have encountered. As times permits, allow participants to discuss the myths.

❖ Focusing on the Word

(About 15 minutes.) Read aloud the introductory para-

graph. Have a volunteer read aloud 1 Samuel 1:1–20. Then discuss the questions that follow.

1. Hannah seems to have experienced four of the five stages of grief—denial, anger, bargaining, and depression. Year after year, Hannah called on the Lord to open her womb. During this time, she was often ridiculed by her rival, Peninnah. This only exasperated her depression. She was so depressed she even lost her appetite (1 Sam. 1:8). She also bargained with the Lord, stating that if the Lord would give her a son, she would give "him to the LORD for all the days of his life" (1 Sam. 1:11). Elkanah was disappointed, perhaps, even depressed over the fact that all Hannah could seemingly think about was her childlessness (1 Sam. 1:8).

2. A childless couple may fear that God is punishing them for an abortion that the woman may have had or the husband may have paid for. They might fear they are being punished because they were involved sexually before marriage.

3. We live in a world where people believe that eventually people get what they deserve. It is, therefore, not unusual for couples struggling with infertility to reason that God is punishing them for something they've done in the past. Read aloud the illustration.

4. Ask the participants to read the Scripture passages to see how childless couples may fear that barrenness is a punishment from God.

a. Jacob acknowledged to Rachel that God was ultimately responsible for the blessing of children (Gen. 30:2).

b. Scripture tells us that upon worshiping the Lord, "Elkanah lay with Hannah his wife, and the Lord remembered her. So in the course of time Hannah conceived and gave birth to a son. She named him Samuel, saying, 'Because I asked the LORD for him.' " (1 Sam. 1:19–20).

c. Children were considered a special blessing for the Jews. It was only through children that their "inheritance," the Promised Land, could be passed on. Children were also considered a blessing because the parents had someone to help them when they did business in "the gate" or to defend when they were being falsely accused (Ps. 127:5). In ancient times, people were dependent on their families for protection and security. Orphans and widows were often scorned or mistreated.

Read aloud the paragraph that states that barrenness is not a punishment for any past or present sin in a Christian's life. God will not use the sins He has forgiven through faith in Jesus as a punishment.

Then discuss the last question.

5. The participants may have found encouragement in knowing that God's faithful people struggled with infertility. As we study these stories, we recognize that these childless couples often experienced the same frustrations that we do in our day and age. Some may even find comfort in the fact that Hannah's persistent praying eventually paid off!

❖ Focusing on My Life

(About 10 minutes.) **1.** Answers will vary. Don't allow this to be a time for the participants to point the finger at each other's spouse. These questions should be answered privately.

2. Let each participant share whether they have heard or made statements similar to the ones given.

3. The sufferer of all sufferers, Job, lost all his property and children. He lost the support of his wife and friends. He even lost his health. His question was simple: "Why God?" God gave His answer in the form of questions: "Where were you when I laid the earth's foundations? Tell me, if you understand. Who marked off its dimensions? Surely you know! Who stretched a measuring line across it?" (Job 38:4–5). The question that's implied in all these questions is, "Job, are you powerful enough to duplicate these acts of God? Are you intelligent enough to run the world?"

4. Ask the participants to circle the stages that best describes them at this time.

Read aloud the next paragraph and the passage from Hebrews.

5. Encourage each participant to choose a person, preferably someone other than his or her spouse, as a prayer partner.

❖ Focusing on the Week Ahead

(About 5 minutes.) Urge participants to complete this activity before the next session. If time permits, provide participants with note cards on which to write the statement. Encourage them to take the card home and to talk to God about the words.

2—Coping

❖ Focusing Our Sights

(About 2 minutes.) Read aloud or have a volunteer read aloud the opening paragraph.

❖ Focusing Our Attention

(About 5 minutes.) Read the introductory paragraph. Then discuss the statements using the questions. Most of the participants will be able to relate to the statements.

❖ Focusing on the Issue

(About 20 minutes.) Read aloud the opening paragraph and the comments shared by support group members. Then ask volunteers to read aloud the different challenges infertile couples must cope with. After each section, give the participants time to answer the questions that follow.

1. Discussing these special celebrations may elicit strong responses from some of the participants. Let the participants brainstorm ways to best handle these special celebrations.

2. Most participants will be able to recall a favorite or disturbing thing people have shared with them about infertility.

3. Don't be surprised at how open people may be in discussing the doctor's workup. Participants may be glad to talk to others who understand what it's like, because they themselves have gone through it.

4. Be especially sensitive to anyone who might be suffering from low self-esteem because of his/her infertility.

5. Ask the participants to work alone for a few moments to jot down other special issues or circumstances they've encountered in their struggle with infertility. Then ask them to compare their list with the others in the group.

❖ Focusing on God's Word

(About 20 minutes.) Ask a volunteer to read aloud 2 Cor. 12:7–9. Then answer the questions that follow.

1. Paul's thorn affected his life greatly. He states that it caused him great "torment."

2. Paul's human weakness provided the ideal opportunity for the display of God's divine power.

3. Answers will vary.

4. Answers will vary. Don't make anyone feel guilty if they say that they feel God's grace hasn't been sufficient.

Ask a volunteer to read aloud Rom. 8:31–32.

5. God "did not spare His own Son, but gave Him up for us all" to take care of our greatest weakness—sin.

6. He will most assuredly also, "along with Him, graciously give us all things" that we need, including help in coping with the anguish of infertility.

❖ Focusing on My Life

(About 5 minutes.) Give participants time to rank the issues. Invite participants to share their ranking. Then invite them to write Rom. 8:32 on an index card you have provided. Urge them to post it in a conspicuous place in their home.

❖ Focusing on the Week Ahead

(About 5 minutes.) Read aloud the final paragraph. Urge participants to review the Scripture passages before the next session.

3—Hoping

❖ Focusing Our Sights

(About 2 minutes.) Invite a volunteer to read aloud the opening paragraph.

Focusing Our Attention

(About 5 minutes.) Read aloud the illustration. Then discuss the questions that follow.

1. The lottery ticket might have given the woman weekly hopes of a better future.

2. Let the participants laugh together about some of the suggestions they've all, at one time or another, received in order to help them conceive.

3. Hope is essential for everything in life, especially for the infertile couple—hope that each new procedure or suggestion might help them have a child.

❖ Focusing on the Issue

(About 20 minutes.) Ask volunteers to read aloud the stories of three couples. Discuss what each couple should do.

❖ Focusing on God's Word

(About 20 minutes.) Read aloud the opening paragraph.

Then invite volunteers to read the selected verses from Gen. 15–21. Invite the participants to answer the questions that follow.

Note. God had promised children to Abraham and Sarah. Although God has made no such promise to the participants in this support-group study, the Bible references that follow can show couples how Abraham and Sarah struggled with their time of waiting and doubt.

1. Abraham and Sarah lived with the problem of infertility. They waited for years to have children but were unable to conceive (Gen. 15:4–5).

2. Abraham was 100 years old. Sarah was 90.

3. Abraham and Sarah both agreed that Abraham should sleep with Hagar, the Egyptian maidservant, and if she conceived, they could build a family through her (Gen. 16:2). Childless couples often go to extraordinary means in order to have children of their own.

4. Abraham and Sarah laughed because they found it hard to believe that at their ages they could still have a child. Though their laughter may have been inexcusable it is understandable, especially by people who have experienced the same infertility problems.

5. Abraham was a man of hope, or assurance, that the things God promised him would be his; "He considered [God] faithful who had made the promise" (Heb. 11:11). He would be the father of "descendants as numerous as the stars in the sky and as countless as the sand on the seashore" (Heb. 11:12). Abraham hoped and believed the promise that God would send a Savior through His seed who would redeem the world (John 8:56).

❖ Focusing on My Life

(About 10 minutes.) **1.** Ask the participants to rank their hope on the continuum. Then ask each participant to explain his or her answer to a partner.

2. Answers will vary. Allow time for participants to share openly.

3. God gives us laughter in order to help us relieve

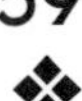

some of our anxiety. Infertile couples need to laugh together.

4. Ask a volunteer to read aloud Is. 40:31–32. Then read the paragraph that follows. Close by praying together the prayer.

❖ Focusing on the Week Ahead

(About 5 minutes.) Provide each participant with an index card on which to write Is. 40:30–31. Ask them to post the card somewhere noticeable.

4—Seeking

❖ Focusing Our Sights

*(About 2 minutes.)*Invite a volunteer to read aloud the opening paragraph.

❖ Focus Our Attention

(About 10 minutes.) Read aloud the first two paragraphs. Then ask the participants whether they agree or disagree with the four statements that follow. The four statements highlight just a few of the many volatile issues that swirl around adoption today. Answers will vary.

❖ Focusing on the Issue

(About 15 minutes.) Ask volunteers to read aloud the common ways childless couples seek to get help for their infertility. Some of the participants may wish to share first-hand information on the treatments they have tried. Then ask the participants to categorize the procedures as acceptable, questionable, or not acceptable.

Christians must remember that the ends do not always justify the means. Despite how much a couple might want a child, Christians needs to measure each procedure against God's Word.

❖ Focusing on God's Word

(About 15 minutes.) Have volunteers read aloud the Scripture passages. Urge participants to underline words and/or phrases that speak to procedures for dealing with infertility. Participants may underline some or all of these words and/or phrases: God commands man and woman to "be fruitful and increase in number" (Gen. 1:28); God initiated and established the one-flesh union described in the words, "a man will leave his father and mother and be united to his wife, and they will become one flesh" (Gen. 2:24); God created us and reminds us that life begins at the time of conception. These biblical concepts will affect our decisions concerning the methods and procedures we might select in order to deal with our infertility.

1. Answer will vary. Most participants will indicate that God created life, desires that man and woman in a one-flesh union "be fruitful," and that life begins at the time of conception.

2. In vitro fertilization is not objectionable if only the sperm and eggs of a man and woman united in the one-flesh union (marriage) are used and that all fertilized eggs are returned to the womb of the mother so they are not destroyed or used for experimentation. Surrogate motherhood may affect the one-flesh union and may cause later difficulties.

3. Read aloud and discuss the quote.

❖ Focusing on My Life

(About 10 minutes.) **1.** Answers will vary. If time permits, let the participants share which factors are most pressing for them.

2. Allow the participants to consider these questions by themselves.

Read aloud the verses from 1 John. Remind participants that God's love for us in Jesus forgives all sins and empowers us to make choices that reflect God's will revealed in His Word.

Pray together the prayer.

❖ Focusing on the Week Ahead

(About 5 minutes.) Read aloud the final paragraph. Urge the participants to spend some time researching infertility at their local library.

5—Moving On

❖ Focusing Our Sights

(About 2 minutes.) Invite a volunteer to read aloud the opening paragraph.

❖ Focusing Our Attention

(About 5 minutes.) Read aloud the opening paragraph and the quotes. Then discuss the questions.

1. Infertility places a physical, psychological, and spiritual strain on a marriage.

2. It is important for couples to eventually close the chapter on infertility because life is often put on hold while the couple tries to have a child.

❖ Focusing on the Issue

*(About 15 minutes.)*Read aloud the opening paragraph. Then ask volunteers to read aloud the different aspects to

consider as people close the chapter on infertility. Allow time for the participants to discuss each issue. Then ask them to list other issues they feel couples need to consider in order to close the chapter.

❖ Focusing on God's Word

*(About 10 minutes.)*Invite a volunteer to read aloud Phil. 3:13–14. Then discuss the questions.

1. St. Paul wisely tells us to forget "what is behind and strain toward what is ahead." Remember all the things St. Paul had to forget? He had at one time persecuted the followers of Christ, sought them out, and witnessed their martyrdom.

2. Jesus "bore our sins in His body on the tree, so that we might die to sins and live for righteousness; by His wounds (we) have been healed" (1 Peter 2:24). He forgives and forgets. So we can forget our past sins.

3. The word *straining* indicates that life, at times, may not be easy.

4. The ultimate "prize" was earned by Jesus Christ for all who believe in Him—eternal life in heaven.

5. The Good News of forgiveness and eternal life through faith in Jesus empowers us to strain toward what is ahead. God promises His faith-strengthening and sustaining power for us in His Word and Sacraments.

6. Answers will vary. Some possible promises include eternal life, forgiveness of sins, strength in trouble, comfort in distress.

❖ Focusing on My Life

(About 10 minutes.) **1.** Answers will vary.

2. Ask a volunteer to read aloud the promise of God found in Ps. 46:1–3.

3. Ask the participants to answer this question individually.

4. One way for a church to help childless couples is to listen to them, perhaps, even provide a support group for them

or set up a surrogate parenting and grandparenting program. It might be difficult emotionally for infertile couples to staff the nursery; however, it certainly depends on each individual couple.

5. Read aloud David's positive action in the face of despair. Then invite a volunteer to read aloud the summary paragraph. Remind participants that David sought strength, hope, and comfort from the Lord in times of distress. God promises to provide us with the same strength, hope, and comfort through His Word.

❖ Focusing on the Week Ahead

(About 5 minutes.) Urge participants to continue caring for one another in the suggested ways. Or have participants suggest others ways they can serve one another.